ALOE VERA
THE HEALTH
AND HEALING PLANT

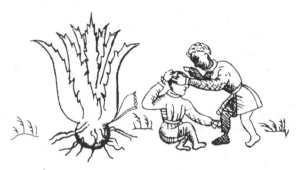

We thank
Steve Brooks, Abel Donnard, Dr. Emile Jaccard,
Jean Moisset, Ernest Schurmann, Denise Spuhler,
Alfred Theodor and Dr. Oskar Zimmermann
for their precious help and counci
in the preparation of this study.
We consulted frequently the book by Bill C. Coats "The Silent Healer"
and "Doctor Aloès" by Robert Dehin.
A short bibliography of the works consulted is included
at the end of this volume.

APOPHTEGME
235, rue du Faubourg Saint-Honoré
75008 PARIS Tél : (1) 42.27.14.89
COPYRIGHT 1995 by Marc Schweizer
All rights reserved
ISBN 2-950853 1-1-0

Ed Maykut and Marc Schweizer

ALOE VERA
The health
and healing plant

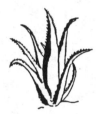

APOPHTEGME

ALOE VERA

THE DOCTOR IN A POT
of CHRISTOPHER COLUMBUS

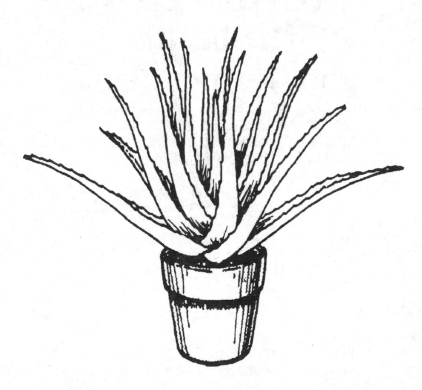

Aloe Vera (Linné) or Aloe barbadensis (Miller)

Introduction

The several thousand year history of the *aloe vera* plant is as fascinating and captivating as a best seller historical novel. Its wild elegance and its therapeutic properties are legend.

In many ancient civilizations it was venerated as a God. In Ancient Egypt aloe was the plant who's blood gave beauty, health and eternity. It took part in the embalming rituals and escorted the Pharaoh on his journey to the other world. For the emperors of mythical China, the healing thorns of the leaf were the sacred nails of the divinities. For the Indians of the Americas, aloe was one of the sixteen plants venerated as Gods. In the great African deserts, the eternal nomades call it the lily of the desert. In North America it is called The Silent Healer and Doctor Aloe. The Russians call it The Elixir* of Longevity.

This rather short book does not have the pretense of offering an exhaustive study of the virtues and powers of aloe. Recent studies have begun to reveal many of them and this magic plant no doubt still has some surprises in reserve for us. It is indeed man's friend par excellence as a healing plant, much as wheat or the olive tree are the nourishing plants.

Today in the USA, in Japan, in Russia and in China aloe has many enthusiastic adepts and followers. In these countries one can find many publications concerning aloe. In France, which was one of the first European countries to recognize the medicinal virtues of the aloe vera plant, the mandarins of medical orthodoxy have hindered the undertaking and publication of serious scientific studies on the subject.

(*) The asterisks refer to the vocabulary page 61.
(1) refer to the numbered notes at the bottom of the page.

Aloe vera

The aloe vera plant named and described by Linne, and the aloe barbadensis plant described by Miller, as well as Lamarck's aloe vulgaris are all one and the same plant. Today, the official botanical classification has retained the name of aloe barbadensis, while the name *aloe vera* has become the popularly used name. We will be using the aloe vera name throughout this book.

Unfortunately there still exists some confusion concerning the plants referred to and described by Linne and Miller. In reality, *aloe vera* and *aloe barbadensis* are the same plant. A detailed description will help dissipate some of the confusion.

Aloe vera grown in fields reaches a height of between 60 to 90 cm. Its plump leaves of 40 to 50 cm in length and 6 to 10 cm wide at the base have small thorns on both edges. The rind or protective layer filters air and water. Under this membrane there is a cellulose dermis covering crystals of calcium oxalate and the pericylic cells of yellow-reddish sap which have laxative properties and are called the blood of aloe. Finally, enclosed in this triple vegetable protection is the colorless parenchyme* which is the much sought after pulp (gel and juice) of the plant. *(see page 34)*. Of course, the quality of this pulp depends a great deal upon the conditions under which it is cultivated, such as the type of soil, the climate and the care.

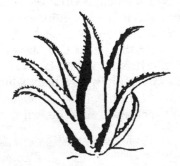

Aloe vera
the health and healing plant

What is the plant ?

The botanists specify that the aloe plant is a phanerogame*
(with flowers) angiosperm*, of the liliacae family. This is
the family of fatty or succulent plants of which cacti are
a part [1].

Its flowers grow on one or several long stems. The flower
resembles a small trumpet, the colors of which range from
greenish white to red passing through yellow and orange. Its
long, thick, and brittle leaves with thorns on both edges grow in
a spiral rosette around a short stem. The mucilage in the
interior of the leaf contains parenchyma, a spongy cellular
structure capable of retaining water filtered by the roots and the
leaf itself. By a complex alchemy (metabolism*) this water is
transformed into a slightly bitter and translucent gel. This is the
gel so prized for its medicinal properties.

The reproduction of the aloe plant can occur in one of two
ways. Birds and insects aid in the pollination of the flowers
which produce seeds. Shoots which grow at the bottom of the
short stem produce new plants.

The aloe plant and its medicinal virtues have been known by
many races and many civilizations around the world. Today,
some overly enthusiastic followers consider it a panacea. We
have taken the name from the greek Aloe, in arabic it is Alloeh,
and in chinese Alo-hei. It is important not to confuse the aloe
plant with the Agave *(see note P16)*, a plant which resembles it
but by botonical classification belongs to amaryllidace family.
There are about 300 species of aloe known in the world and

*(1) The aloe vera plant is a member of the liliacae family as are the hyacinth,
lily, tulip, asparagas, garlic and onion.*

7

new ones are discovered every year. They include small plants of a few centimeters to tree-like aloe dozens of meters high. But few of these species are medicinal. The aloe plant most used in medicine is the aloe vera. These are the aloes from: the island of Socotra (aloe succotrina), Cape aloe (aloe africana), aloe saponaria, aloe sinensis, aloe arborscens, aloe Natal; and aloe ferox with its extra sharp thorns.

The aloe plant grows naturally in most tropical and subtropical regions. Some species are used to produce ropes and until the appearance of synthetic fibers, they provided a natural rot proof material used in the manufacture of marine cords. It still has wide use in many parts of the world for this and many other applications such as the fabrication of mats and cloth requiring a resistant material.

Aloe ferox and aloe saponara are used extensively by the Japanese. Aloe arborescens is the one studied by Russian researchers (see below). The tree-like aloe excelsa of Zimbabwe reaches more than ten meters in height.

But, it is essentially the pulp contained in the long meaty leaves of the aloe barbadensis , the aloe vera of Linne *(see P6)* that is found in many beauty (cosmetic) products and is used for its medicinal virtues to heal many ills and wounds. Is the rapid and widespread development of its paramedical use observed in recent years just a passing fancy? Or is it really a result of the many known and some unknown qualities attributed to aloe vera? Indeed, in studying its history and recent developments, we are forced to admit that in spite of an enigmatic appearance, this unusual plant has, and still hides, many rich virtues, and it is ready to share them with us.

A small experiment

To demonstrate the surprising capacity for survival of the aloe vera plant we suggest the following experiment :

Cut a leaf from the plant at its base. At first you will notice the appearance of a gentle oozing of juice at the cut. Then, within a few minutes it stops and a skin begins to cover it.

The plant has healed itself!

Redo the experiment on a freshly cut leaf which you have kept in the refrigerator for ten days. Make an incision and you will note the same self healing (regenerating) process occur. An aloe plant uprooted and abandoned in the hot sun will resist for a month and will retain its vital powers intact.

Universal acceptance and reputation

Aloe vera has been known for its many qualities on all five continents. The Europeans were happy to limit its use until recently in the form of a dry powdered extract, only as a bitter laxative and a vermifuge. They had not developed a method to stabilize and preserve the virtues of the gel.

Today, the proofs exist that the fresh and stabilized gel of the leaf heal everyday minor domestic injuries and problems such as: burns, cuts, insect bites, digestive problems, eczema, etc. It is known to be an excellent wound healer, and when drunk in the form of a juice as a nutritional complement, it is tonic and stimulating.

For many years, many athletes have been using aloe to treat sprains, tendinitis, and other wounds associated with their sports. Some athletes drink the juice of aloe as a natural stimulant which is not detectable during an anti-drug control.

Women use it in rejuvenating creams, in face masks, shampoos, hair lotions, etc. Some say that there is nothing better as a basic treatment for hepatitis, asthma, leprosy, and skin diseases. In brief, it is par excellence the first aid plant.

You are a enclosed garden,
my sister, my fiancée:
There is under your tongue
milk and honey.
And the odor of your clothes
is like the odor of Lebanon.
You are as a flower garden,
a perfumed spring,
a sealed fountain.
Your waters feed a delightful
rose garden where grow trees
with fruits of gold and purple,
The mango and pomegranate
with their delicious fruits.
The privet with the nard
and saffron
The aromatic reed
and the cinnamon,
And all the trees which give
incense, myrrh and aloe...

Song of Songs

THE MARVELOUS HISTORY OF ALOE

Antiquity

The healing values of aloe have been known since antiquity. Authentic witnesses and legendary stories abound in the history of antiquity. The first written reference to the therapeutic use of aloe mussabar is found on clay tablets dating from the reign of the Sumarian king, Akkad. The aloe plant is shown on painted vases dating from archaic times. The Egyptian book of remedies found in the famous Ebers papyrus (XV century BC) also mention aloe in healing formulas which probably existed 3000 years before our time. For the Hindus, aloe holds an important position among the secret plants of Atharvaveda [2] where it was already known as the *"silent healer"*. In the old testament we find references to aloe in the sacred books *(Numbers, The Song of Songs)*.

In the new testament we find this reference in "The Gospel According to Saint John" : *"And there came also Nicodemus who at the first came to Jesus at night, and brought a mixture of myrrh and aloe. They then took the body of Jesus and bound it in linen cloth along with spices, as is the burial custom of the Jews"*.

During the long period of persecution of the Christians by the Romans, the Romans forced the Christians to burn incense as an offering to their Gods. To circumvent this obligation, which they detested, certain christian communities belonging to the primitive church (Edesse) replaced the officially imposed incense prepared from the aquilaire agaloche (aloe wood) by a sacred incense made from biblical aloe mixed with myrrh and benzoin.[3] *Nota page 12.*

(2) Atharvaveda : one of the four Veda (in Sanskrit: knowledge) which are fundamental texts of Hinduism containing formulas and incantations. It is composed of about 731 hymns including about 6000 verses, prayers, expiatories, magic incantations, spells, secret plants and preparations for the treatment of all sorts of illnesses. Completed by the Ayuveda (Veda-life) the Hindu science of medicine.

11

Ancient Egypt

In ancient Egypt aloe had the reputation of being able to keep women young and beautiful. The Pharaohs considered it to be an elixir of long life. It was a tradition to offer an aloe plant as a symbol of eternal life during the funeral ceremonies. Planted along the route leading to the "Valley of the Kings" and around the pyramids, the aloe accompanied the Pharaohs to the beyond. It served to nourish and heal him during the long journey. When the plant was in flower, it was a sign that the deceased had reached his destination. The priests also used the plant in their funeral rites and incorporated it into their embalming formulas under the name of "the plant of immortality".

The ancien Egyptians also appreciated aloe for its virtues as a cosmetic. According to legend, the beauty of the skin and eyes of Cleopatra owed a lot to lotions containing aloe made by one of her Nubian slaves. The legendary beauty of Queen Nephertiti are said to be the result of her baths in mare's milk and aloe pulp.

Greek and Roman

For the ancient greeks aloe symbolized beauty, patience, fortune, and health. Hippocratus, in one of his treatises, described some of the healing properties of aloe: growth of hair, healing of tumors, relief from dysentery and stomach pains. It is said that about 330 B.C. Alexander the Great was wounded by an enemy arrow during his siege of Gaza (Palestine). As he continued his conquering cavalcade through Egypt and the desert of Tipoli, the wound became infected and would not heal. During his stopover at the Oasis of Amon he was proclaimed son of the God Zeus. At this time his private tutor, the famous Aristotle, sent a priest with an oil made from the aloe plant grown on the island of Socotra. The priest treated the wound of Alexender which soon healed. It is also said that it was Aristotle who incited Alexander to mount a naval

(3) *There is often some confusion in ancient writings concerning the difference between the aloe leaf and aloe wood. The aloe wood comes from a tree (Aguilaria Agalogus) the aromatic wood of which is used to make incense.*

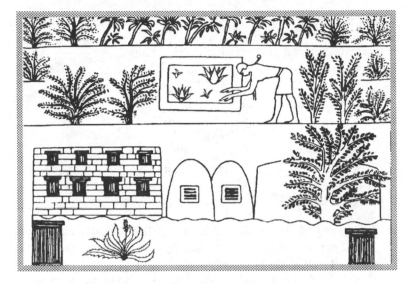

expedition to conquer the island of Socotra and take possession of the aloe plantations. It was said that the juice of the aloe plant rendered the warriors invulnerable.

For many peoples of the Middle East, the juice of aloe had the reputation of bringing wisdom and immortality. The Phoenicians dried the pulp extracted from the leaves, packed the powder in goat skins and exported it westward to the greco-roman world.

It was during the punic wars in North Africa that the Romans discovered the healing virtues of aloe. They discovered, to their great astonishment, that their Carthaginian prisoners used great quantities of the juice of aloe to heal their wounds.

During the first century A.D. Celcius, one of the precursors of roman medecine, vaunted the virtues of aloe. As for Dioscoride who had served for many years with the roman armies, he described with great enthusiasm in his De Materia Medica the many healing properties of aloe, among which he included its virtues of : coagulating the blood of bleeding wounds, healing of scratches and open wounds, healing of boils and hemorrhoids. He also claimed that treatment with the fresh pulp stopped the falling of hair and healed eye infections.

13

In his famous book of natural history, Pline the Ancient (23-79 A.B.) describes a novel way of curing dysentery, which was the injection of the juice of aloe into the colon.

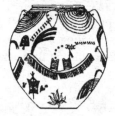

Africa and the Orient

Since ancient times, the Bedouins of the Arabian Peninsula and the Tuareg warriors of the Sahara know well the virtues of aloe which they call the "Desert Lily".

To protect their homes against all sorts of evil, the inhabitants of Mesopotemia decorated their doors with the leaves of aloe.

During the time of an epidemic or famine, the Parthes and the Scythes ate the pulp of the aloe.

The island of Socotra in the Indian ocean was renowned for its plantations of medicinal aloe as early as the fifth century before Christ. The merchants of the island exported their aloe (Mussabar) as far as China as *alo-hei*. On the route they traded with India, Malaysia and Tibet.

Initiation to the medicinal virtues and the power of aloe and hemp were part of the teachings of the Ismaelian sect. One of the first and best known representatives was doctor and philosopher Avicenne who had inspired Hassan ihn al-Sabbah, the famous *"Old man of the mountain"* chief of the Brotherhood of Assassins.

Their doctrine included the teaching by degree of all the mysteries of the "seven Sabayah" or the "Path of Knowledge" by which their adepts could acquire magic powers. Aloe, which was grown, along with hemp, around the fortress of Alamut (northern Persia) was considered by the Ismaelians to be a protector, an antidote, and an elixir of long life. It is said that one of the secrets of the longevity of the Templar Knights resided in the famous *"Elixir of Jerusalem"* composed of a mixture of the pulp of aloe, hemp, and palm wine.

Eight centuries later, Dominique Larry, a chief surgeon with Napoleon's army in Egypt, learned of the virtues of aloe when he witnessed the miraculous healing of the most terrible wounds of his Mamalouks by a Marabout. He then used his saber to cut the leaves of the aloe plant to treat the famous Grognards of the *Grand Armé*e. This is the origin of the expression: *"sabrer l'aloès"* (archives of the Val de Grace hospital).

Hindu Ayurvedic [4] medicine has always held aloe in high esteem as an integral part of its pharmacopoeia. It was considered to be a sacred plant, was used in certain sacrificial rituals , and certain species were rigorously protected. Even today, in modern India, aloe leaves are placed upon funeral pyres as symbols of rebirth and eternity.

The Middle Ages and Renaissance

In the famous medical texts of the school of Salerno, Constantin the Africain and his disciples gave high marks to the therapeutic virtues of aloe. In his book entitled *"Doctor Aloe"*, Robert Dehin, cited earlier (see bibliography), included this famous poem dedicated to this fetish plant :

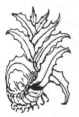

It dries a wound, it revives the flesh,
In diseased foreskin, it destroys the cancer,
It purges the secretion of the eye, it clears
The head, the blocked ear and the coated tongue.
The sickly stomach it revives the vigor,
Stops the fall of hair, and gives it life.
It relieves the liver and heals icterus.

It was during the Crusades that the christian warriors from the west discovered the virtues of aloe. Their moslem adversaries considered it to be their remedy par excellence. During their westward conquests, the Arabs introduced the aloe into Spain.

(4) Ayurveda or Veda of life. Traditional Hindu medicine whose recipes and formulas are part of the Athervaveda. See page 11.

It was the pulp of aloe which saved many of the spanish sailors on the Santa Maria from disease and malnutrition and inspired Columbus to call it the *"doctor in a pot"*. After Columbus, all the spanish ships carried aloe.

Paracelse, the famous renaissance doctor, discovered the merits of aloe in Salerno, Italy and later during his travels in Portugal and Spain. In a letter to Amberg he praised aloe in the following terms : *"The secret and mysterious aloe who's golden juice heals burns and blood poisoning"*. But it was the portuguese and spanish Jesuit missionaries who followed the first explorers who introduced the cultivation of aloe in America, Africa and the Far East. For they knew well the many healing properties of the aloe plant. The Indians they converted called the plant : *"The Tree of Jesus"*.

The American Indians

The aloe plant, along with the Agave[5] was one of the sixteen plants considered sacred by the American Indians. But there existed a confusion between the two even though they are not of the same botanical family and do not have the same properties.

The Indians ate the leaves of aloe after cooking them over hot ashes, and used the pulp to stop hemorrhages and heal wounds. The bitter fermented juice of aloe was used to calm the stomach, to flush the kidneys and the bladder, to dissolve kidney stones, cure coughs, relieve chest pains, and to bring on menstruation.

In pre-colombian America, the young Maya women used aloe juice as a cosmetic, much like Cleopatra, to attract the young men. Before leaving for battle or on a hunt the warriors rubbed their bodies with aloe pulp. A curious Maya tradition claimed that if the pulque (agave wine) brought on madness, on

---

(5) *Agave (from agauos, magnificent). A plant of the amaryllidacae family, often confused with aloe and especially with aloe vera who's flower is also yellow. The agave of Mexico was a sacred plant of the indians, especially of the Mayas and the Tolteques.*
The leaves are used to make sisal, a vegetable fiber, and the juice a wine called pulpec, this wine is distilled to produce Mescal and Tequila. The floral stem of the agave can grow to a height of 12 meters but it produces seeds only once in its long life.

16

the contrary the wine of aloe cured madness. The Jivaros had named it "the heavenly doctor" because they believed the sacred plant made them invulnerable.

The Mazahuas tribes considered aloe as a magic plant which cured all the ills of he who ate it, gave him great power *"by entering God into him"*, and clarified the spirit of the insane, the drunkard and the deranged. They cured migraine headaches by applying a poultice of aloe around the aching head. The Tictle or healer of the Nahua tribes was a bit of a witch doctor who knew which plants had the magic power to heal. He healed wounds, and insect and snake bites by covering the wounds and bites with the *"blood"* of aloe. Yet it was the Jesuit missionaries who really popularized the use of aloe as a healer in the Spanish American colonies. For they had learned all of its medicinal virtues in Spain.

The Far East

In Japan aloe is an extremely popular plant. Hundreds of species are cultivated for multiple uses. It is eaten and drunk. It is used in many forms to treat and heal. In ancient times, the Samurai smeared their bodies with the pulp of aloe to chase away the demons and to render themselves immortal. Today, the pulp of *aloe saponaria* is used to make cosmetics and soap. *Aloe ferox, aloe thraskii* and *aloe marlothii* enter into the composition of numerous pharmaceutical and cosmetic products.

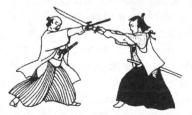

The Chinese are as fond of aloe as their Japanese cousins and use it in many forms. For centuries aloe has been used specifically to treat burns and ailments of the skin. The pharmacopoea of Li Shih-Shen (1518-1593) cites *aloe* as one

17

of the plants with major therapeutic virtues and calls it: *"the harmonic remedy"*.

The spines of *aloe ferox* were used as acupuncture needles by the famous *"bare foot doctors"*, the itinerant therapists. Traditional chinese medical practice has always been very precise in the formulation of its prescriptions and the rules to follow.

The phase of the moon, the height of the sun above the horizon and the time of day were all taken into account. These rules are applied even today by many chinese doctors. Modern chinese medicine uses the pulp of *aloe sinensis* in the treatment of arteriosclerosis.

From Legend to Science

In many countries where modern occidental medicine has not replaced tradition medical practice, aloe remains the medicinal plant par excellence. Local traditions attribute to this magic plant the virtues of a protector and a good luck charm. Moslums returning from their pilgrimage hang aloe leaves over their doors as a proof of their pilgrimage and as an invitation to the Prophet to return their visit. The Africaners and the Zoulous also consider the plant to be a cure-all. Certain desert peoples smear their bodies and hair with a soap made from the juice of aloe which gives them a radiant skin and abundant and luxuriant hair.

Carol Miller Kent, in her book : *Aloe Vera*, claims that a salve made of aloe was part of the medicines on board the capsule which landed on the moon in 1969. The work of the Soviet biologist Israel Brekhman, classified secret for a long time, prove the effectiveness of aloe in the treatment of nuclear radiation. It was Brekhman who coined the term "adaptogene" to explain the regulatory effect of aloe on the organism.

The thousand year reputation of aloe and the renown of its legendary virtues has prompted innumerable scientists to study its medicinal properties and therapeutic effects. In spite of their bias against this *"old ladies remedy"* they had to admit, not without surprise, that many of the legendary virtues of aloe were not just imaginary. In fact, they have discovered new and unknown virtues.

THE PIONEERS OF MODERN RESEARCH

American Research

In 1851 Smith and Stenhouse were the first to identify the principle active substance of aloe which they named "Aloin*" *(6)*.

In 1912, H.W. Johnstone, a plantation owner in Kentucky, observed with surprise the healing powers of aloe when some of his plantation workers were badly burned during a fire. The mammys had covered their burns with the pulp of aloe. He then decided to cultivate the plant and to market the pulp in the form of a salve.

During the 1930's, Creston Collins and his son tested the virtues of aloe scientifically and proved its efficiency as a healing agent. In a celebrated report they confirmed the ability of aloe vera (barbadensis) to heal the burns caused by radiotherapy.

After their publication, several researchers began to study the chemical composition of the plant. In 1938 Chopia and Gosh identified some of its principal active elements : aloin, emodine, chysophanic acid, resin gum, and traces of volatile and non-volatile oils.

In 1942, Rodney M. Stockton, a chemical engineer, while in Florida on vacation suffered a severe sunburn. Some friends covered the burned area with the gel-like pulp taken from the leaves of a fresh aloe vera plant. Stockton was surprised when the pain stopped almost immediately. He was also so impressed by the rapidity of the healing, that he decided to study the plant more closely. In 1947 he moved to Florida and did a lot of experimenting to see if the phenomena were scientifically

---

(6) Aloin : during the nineteenth century, european medicine knew aloe essentially for its use as a purgative attributed to the action of aloin contained in the skin of the plant. Only the empiricists in the coutries where aloe vera was grown used the fresh translucent pulp extracted from the leaf..

reproductive. He found that they were. He then worked on a method of stabilizing the gel of the plant and was able to develop an aloe based salve as a treatment for burns. The product became popular for some time after being vaunted on a popular TV show.

In the late 1950's Bill C. Coats, a Texas pharmacist who had passed many years studying the plant, finally succeeded in developing a stabilized version of the fresh pulp (gel). The degradation of the fresh pulp had always been a major obstacle to its successful commercialization. His secret process of stabilization, a perfectly natural but rather complicated one, was patented. It consists of incubating the pulp at different temperatures for three days then adding vitamins C and E plus sorbitol, all of which are efficient anti-oxidizers.

This major discovery finally permitted the commercialization of a reliable line of products which have gradually conquered the world. Bill Coats published several books in the early 1980's in which he explains in detail the results of his research and efforts to make the healing virtues of the aloe vera plant known and available to all. *(See : Culture and Transformation of Aloe P 27 and the bibliography P 62).*

New Discoveries

During the previous ten years, research concerning the composition and properties of aloe vera has been intense and has progressed rapidly. In 1984 studies under the direction of Ivan E. Danhof, professor of physiology at the University of Texas and chief of the *Research Laboratory of North Texas*, revealed that the application of aloe gel on the skin accelerated 6 to 8 times the natural rate of production of fibroblasts*. The fibroblasts are responsible for the fabrication of collogen the protein which controls the aging process of the skin and the formation of wrinkles. According to Danhof it is the presence of the poly-saccharides in the aloe gel which facilitate the reorganization of the cells of the thin protective outer layer of the skin. He also demonstrated the fantastic moisturizing capacity of the gel of aloe (95% water), that is 3 to 4 times faster than ordinary water.

It is thanks to the works of Fujita, a japanese doctor, that we owe the discovery that it is the enzyme* bradykinase along with salisylic acide, both contained in the aloe gel, which give it the remarkable pain killing and healing properties. *(See P31 +)*.

In 1985, doctor Bill McAnalley isolated a polysaccharide from aloe vera (barbadensis) called acemannon which he named *carrisyn* [7]. About the same time researchers in Canada isolated the molecule acemannon which seemed to possess remarkable anti-viral properties. Since, clinical trials on AIDES patients have shown that carrisyn re-enforces the natural defense system of the patient and thus stops the progression of the HIV virus. This result has been corroborated by the studies of several other researchers, notably by doctor Reg McDaniel who emphasizes that contrary to most other treatments, the one based upon carrisyn produced no negative side effects. The announcement, of course, was sensational.

Doctor McDaniel stated : *"It appears that carrisyn neutralizes the virus by transforming it's protein envelope thus preventing it from attaching itself to the T4 cells (preliminary* report published in 1987 in the magazine *Clinical Review)*.

Carrington Laboratories have obtained the authorization from the FDA (Food and Drug Administration) to experiment carrisyn on human patients. Preliminary results appear to be encouraging.

(7) Carrisyn is the commercial name of acemannon patented by Carrington Laboratories.

During the same period, scientists of the now defunct URSS had also been at work. Professor Brekhman (cited above), the ophtalmologist Vladimir Filatov and the neurologist Serge Pavlenko, just to mention a few, studied the surprising virtues of medicinal aloe.

Wolfgang Wirth in his book *"Heal with Aloe"* recounts this epic, which we summarize below.

The Secrets of Russian Aloe

Professor Vladimir Filatov (2/28/75-10/30/56) an eminent ophthalmologist from Odessa and a specialist in tissue grafting was one of the modern pioneers in the therapeutic use of aloe. Filatov was a dynamic researcher and by nature very curious. He was not one to be content with the narrow paths of official medical practice. His motto was: *"he who is right is the one who heals"*.

Without apriority and dogmatism, this brilliant surgeon and researcher studied different non-orthodox therapies which his peers considered to be superstitious magic. He studied homeopathy, naturopathy, energies, was a militant for unitary medicine, and had a holistic view of man and illnesses. For him chemotherapy and healing with plants had the same value and they should be practiced together rather than be opposed in sterile controversy.

He had the habit of saying: *"In the case where one method does not work, another should be tried! For every illness there is a cure. It is up to us, the doctors, to discover the cure !"*

In his many travels through the Caucasus and Siberia he was always on the lookout for medicinal plants and the secrets of the local healers.

After the October revolution, Filatov was able to continue his research under the restrictive soviet regime without too much difficulty by maliciously naming his method *"dialectic medicine"*.

Thus, the political commissars and the mandarins of official soviet medicine allowed him to work in peace.

Filatov considered that the opposition between the empirical healer and allopathic medicine was a false problem. He preferred to teach the healers at least the rudiments of modern medical science and to introduce into the medical schools a more open approach to the virtues and practices of traditional folk medicine. In this way he knew that both would benefit.

Filatov was the pioneer of Keratoplasty (cornea grafting). The principle discovery of Filatov was that by transplanting (grafting) a small fragment of live healthy cornea tissue on the cornea having become opaque because of a cataract, the opaque cornea refound its original transparency. He also noted that this process was even more rapid when he used a fragment of cornea which had been extracted from a corpse and refrigerated at 2 degrees centigrade for a short time. Using his method, Filatov was able to cure thousands of cases of cataract and of keratoscleritus caused by syphilis. Intrigued by the fact that the grafts taken from a corpse and refrigerated seemed to be more effective than the grafts taken from a living cornea, he turned his research toward this seemingly strange reaction. What he found was that tissue of this type, when properly taken and refrigerated, continued to live and to manufacture active substances specifically intended to combat traumatisms. Thus, a tiny graft of tissue obtained from a dead body was able to

regenerate diseased tissue of a living body. Suspecting that it must be due to substances contained in the cells, Filatov named them *"biogenic stimulators"*. Filatov also spent a considerable amount of his time studying plants. At first he studied ginseng, the divine plant. Later, after having observed the surprising cures obtained by the traditional healers of Central Asia, he studed aloe (aloe arborescens) abundant in the southern parts of the USSR.

He continued his research with plants to see if his theory on biogenic stimulators could also be applied to plants and, after hundreds of successful experiments with aloe, he developed the following technique :

He cut leaves of *aloe arborescens* and refrigerated them at 2 degrees centigrade for 10 days. He then extracted some pulp from these leaves and injected it under the skin of his patients. He observed the same curative effects as with the transplants of tissue obtained from a corpse !

From his experimental results, Filatov arrived at the following hypothesis: *"all sudden deterioration in the life of an animal or vegetable organism provokes in the organism the secretion of biogenic stimulators, vital regulators with truly astounding therapeutic properties"*.

He also noted to his great surprise, that the same leaves of aloe, when exposed in an autoclave at a temperature of 120 degrees centigrade, retained some of their properties even though their enzymes had been destroyed.

Filatov concluded that it was not the tissue of the cornea itself or the pulp of aloe which initiated the healing process, but that it was the biogenic stimulators they contained.

Although he was able to affirm their healing effects, Filatov was not able to explain what the biogenic stimulators were or how they functioned.

Based upon his principle that *"he who heals is right"*, Filatov treated innumerable patients with preparations based upon aloe (biostimulated aloe). He noted that the plant stimulated certain physiological functions of the organism and augmented considerably the immunity defenses.

It was doctor Max Brandt who attempted to explain this process scientifically: *"the mechanism by which the biogenic stimulators of aloe function is via the central nervous system. If aloe provokes an increase in the duration of conditioned reflexes, it induces a gradual decrease in their power arriving finally at their complete disappearance. We can therefore speak of the reinforcement of the inhibition process of the central nervous system as already described by Pavlov.*

The slowing down of activity of the cerebral cortex produced by the aloe is considered by many renowned researchers to be a therapeutic protector. (...) All clinical data available demonstrate the significant biological activity of aloe and a definite effect of the biogenic stimulators on the central nervous system." [8]

After the death of Filatov, several of his students continued his work. Doctor Woljanski studied and developed a method using aloe by which he was able to heal even some of the most recalcitrant cases of sciatica, and doctor Kurako had obtained excellent results in treating cases of inflammation of the spinal cord.

In geriatrics, doctor Kalmanovicz was able to note a decrease in the phenomena of asthenia and a remarkable increase in the intellectual capacity of the aged patients he treated with aloe.

According to doctor Brandt the discovery of biogenic stimulators [8] by Filatov now furnished the missing proof of the effectiveness of the therapeutic treatments which are an integral part of traditional medicine in numerous countries.

According to doctor Brandt a therapy based upon aloe can be considered now as an important part of biological medicine. Aloe is effective in treating diseases of the eyes. It improves and stabilizes visual capacity. It relieves and in some cases cures asthma. It has a positive influence upon all diseases which are associated with the immunity system such as: cancer, AIDS and multiple sclerosis. It improves measurably the quality of life of the aged. It's effectiveness against common and radiation burns is common knowledge.

The active agents in aloe correspond to the micro elements of our bodies, thus they compensate deficits which may occur.

(8) Wirth : Heal with Aloe, Edition Wilhelm Ensthaler.

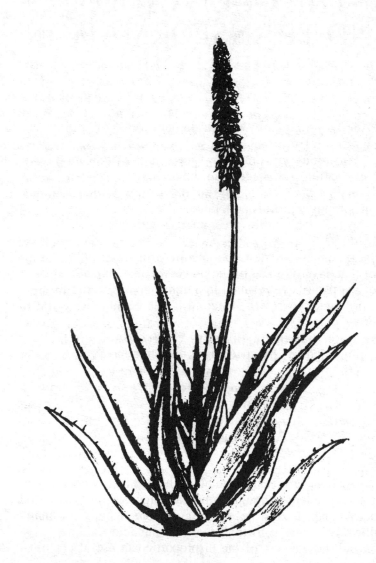

Laurence Tual : Aloe vera

THE CULTIVATION
AND TRANSFORMATION
OF ALOE

The aloe plant grows wild in semi-desert regions with warm climates. It grows best on dry, sandy and calcareous terrain. *Aloe vera* (the principal medicinal species), called the vegetable doctor by the Americans, is relatively easy to grow. The plants are grown naturally in regions propitious for its cultivation.

Today the plant is grown commercially in many countries of the world [9].

The discovery of new therapeutic properties of the plant (other than laxative) and of the processes of stabilization of the gel of the plant have resulted in a tremendous demand for aloe vera products. In North America it has become a veritable boom.

We note that in our modern civilization, where bio-technology and overly specialised medicine have replaced the

often excellent services of the old fashioned family doctor with his often excellent although empirical diagnosis, this secret and seductive plant is fast becoming a welcome member of many families. By using it to treat many of our minor ailments we can avoid the dangers of the disproportionate use of chemical medicines.

(9) Aloe vera of America, a Texas company, is the largest producer and processor of aloe vera in the word today (75 % of the market.)

It is a widely know fact that the most effective treatment is with the gel taken from a fresh leaf. However, in temperate climates it is rather difficult to grow the plant in a garden or in an apartment, since it is a tropical plant. Fortunately, today there are prepared aloe vera products on the market which are perfectly natural and of good quality, and which perform as well as the fresh leaf-gel.

Manufacturing of Extracts of Aloe Vera

The processes for the manufacture of the medicinal extracts of the aloe plant have evolved over the centuries. Years ago, the Arabs placed the pulp extracted from the leaves in sacks made of goat skin and allowed it to dry in the hot sun to produce a resinous powder. The residents of the island of Socotrin also dried it in the sun to produce a powder, while the settlers of Jamaica boiled the leaves to produce a concentrate of the juice. The slaves of the island of Barbados cut the leaves and collected the juice in a wooden receptacle then boiled the juice to produce a sugar-like powder.

Today, even though the manual harvesting and preparation of the leaves is still practiced in some countries, in the western world there now exist large companies specialized in the cultivation and processing of aloe vera using modern machines and methods to insure the quality of the products.

When the Americans learned that it was the gel of the leaf which contained the majority of active elements of the plant, they developed semi-automatic methods of extraction of the pulp thus avoiding the presence of aloin [10] and several other chemicals and undesirable substances in the medicinal gel.

But, the key to a good aloe gel does not depend only upon the method of extraction. What is of prime importance is the method and the efficiency of stabilization to insure proper

[10] *We must note that there is a difference between the thin layer of yellowish sap under the outer rind of the leaf of aloe vera which contains the aloin, and the translucent gel which forms the inner pulp.*

conservation of the final product.

Today, to satisfy the large demand, the aloe vera vera plants are grown on large plantations, especially in south Texas and Mexico. At the age of 4 or 5 years, the leaves reach maturity and weigh between 2 and 3 pounds. They are cut carefully at the base by the field hands and transported immediately to the nearby processing plant. The are never exposed to the burning sun where they would degenerate rapidly.

At the factory they are first treated in a disenfectant solution to wash off the dust and dirt, and to kill the bacteria and fungus. They are then sorted according to size and once again brushed and rinced to insure absolute cleanliness. Now, they are ready for the extraction of the interior gel by machine.

There exist two types of machines to accomplish this extraction. The oldest type, called the "Thompson fillet machine", ressembles an old fashioned washing machine ringer. The gel is literally squeezed from the leaf. The latest and most ingenious machine peals off the bottom and top rind of the leaf to expose the pure interior gel of the leaf, thus avoiding the extraction of the undesired aloin and parts of the rind with the gel; It is this gel which is then treated by special, patented, processes to produce a stabilized gel, that is, one able to retain its beneficial and curative properties intact over a long period of time. This gel is then processed to produce the many different aloe vera products we find on the world market today.

Conservation

The whitish translucent gel of the leaf of the aloe vera plant once extracted is very unstable. Left at normal temperatures it oxidizes rapidly and loses most of its therapeutic properties. Even when placed in a refrigerator it is altered in a few days. This is the reason why the veritable problem of its successful commercialization was to develop a reliable means of stabilization.

In their first attempts, researchers exposed the pulp to utraviolet radiation. This process was quickly abandoned because it modified the chemical composition of the pulp.

Others tried pasteurization by heating the pulp at 60 degrees centigrade after having added hydrogen peroxyde. This method was also unsuccessful.

Others used a freeze-drying method. The results were fairly good since the rehydrated pulp seemed to retain its properties.

Others tried dehydration at medium to high temperatures. Still others tried irradiation but soon abandoned the technique.

In any case, none of the above methods were able to successfully preserve the natural properties of the fresh pulp, especially the vitamins and enzymes which are the active elements of the aloe pulp. So, the problem was to find a method of conservation/stabilization which did not destroy the enzymes and the vitamins.

It was Bill Coats, the founder of the company Aloe Vera of America (AVA) who developed and patented a viable technique of conservation which appears to be the best available to this day. It consists of incubating the pulp in tanks after having added vitamin C (ascorbic acid), vitamin E (tocopherol), and sorbitol to prevent oxidation. By controlling the process at precise temperatures[11], he was able to obtain a chemical reaction which conserved the product.

(11) *These temperatures have not been disclosed, but they do not damage the medicinal integrity of the pulp.*

MEDICINAL PROPERTIES

Let is recall that in most so called advanced countries, a new medication or a new product based upon plant extracts are approved by official authorities only if the exact chemical composition is known. Thus, a plant such as aloe which has proven itself over the centuries and has been an integral part of the pharmacopeoia of traditional folk healers and herbalists, will not be officially recognized until it has passed all the obstacles of experimental protocols. When we add to this obstacle, the ferocious competitive war being fought in the shadow of the giant pharmaceutical laboratories, we may better understand why the enormous financial interests manage to retard or stop the open sale of excellent natural products which are often much cheaper.

It becomes obvious that a plant, which can be easily grown in a desert, in a field, in a garden or on a balcony and has the capacity of healing numerous injuries and illnesses, can cause confusion in the controlled panorama of big international Medical Business !

One of the first prepared products of aloe was a powder produced from the dried leaves. In the countries where this powder was produced, the reddish sap just under the outer rind was also used as a medicine. These products are still manufactured and used in the islands of the West Indies and other underdeveloped countries. A stabilized form of the pulp of aloe permitting a wide distribution and prolonged use of the product was not available until after the 1960's. Today, it is the stabilized gel of the aloe vera plant which is in wide use.

The ancients considered aloe an elixir of long life but very few understood the difference between the yellow red sap layer just under the rind of the leaf and the colorless gel in the plump heart of the leaf. The aloin contained in the pericyclic cells of the aloe sap is: cholagogic, stomachic, laxative, and purgative. But it is the pulp which is the most active part of the plant. It is : astringent*, bactericidal*, sedative, healing, fungicidal*, anti-inflammatory*, haemostatic*, and virucidal*. It is known for its ability to: anaesthetize tissues, stop itching, and relieve insect bites. It also lowers fevers, combats constipation, dilates the capillary vessels, and purifys the blood. In dermatology, the gel of aloe revitalizes the skin tissues, digests the dead cells, moisturizes dry skin and penetrates the dermis* easily to bring its healing benefits.

There is an uncanny relationship between the rind and the gel of the aloe vera leaf when used as an applique in poultices and wraps in the treatment of burns, wounds, and insect bites.

During the past half century, researchers have enriched the already long list of traditional aloe properties with some interesting new functions. Taken internally, the pulp of aloe vera has been proven to be an excellent biological regulator and an immuno-stimulator. Certain American doctors even report having obtained good results in treating cancer and AIDS.

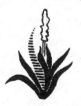

The richness of aloe pulp in vitamins, minerals and other nutritive substances has also convinced many that it is an excellent food supplement.

In spite of all the folklore and new findings, we must be prudent. Isn't aloe's reputation as a miraculous plant,and all those praises and claims, just folk legends? Or isn't it just a vulgar publicity campaign to promote the sale of the hundreds of more or less effective products now being offered on the market throughout the world ?

What argues most convincingly in favor of the intrinsic virtues of aloe, is that it has been adopted and widely used over the centuries by diverse peoples living as far apart from each other as: ancient Egypt, India, pre-columbian America, Madagascar, primitive Australia, etc.

It is obvious that this somewhat "magic" reputation surrounding the virtues of aloe is repulsive to many scientists. The same who have a strong tendency to discredit alternate natural medical practice and deny the efficacy of natural therapeutics, which they qualify as merely placebos*.

However, this has not stopped a great number of doctors, pharmacists, and biologists from undertaking serious studies of aloe and presenting results which confirm the legendary medicinal properties of aloe. Even better, they have discovered new virtues, such as its nutritive values. The pulp extracted from the leaves has been found to be rich in minerals, vitamins, and many other nutritive elements.

The basic problem is that the pulp contained in the long meaty leaves of aloe vera oxidize rapidly upon contact with air and the resulting degradation destroys most of its active elements. As we have already explained above, to conserve the pulp the ancients dried it and produced a powder. This has been replaced in modern times with much more effective and efficient methods which conserve all its native powers.

Cross section of a leaf of *aloe vera*

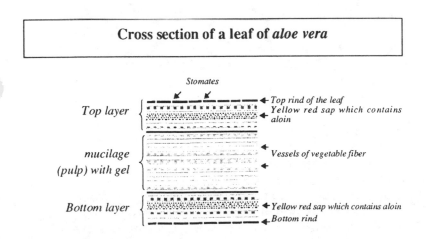

Stomates

Top layer {
— Top rind of the leaf
Yellow red sap which contains aloin

mucilage (pulp) with gel {
— Vessels of vegetable fiber

Bottom layer {
Yellow red sap which contains aloin
Bottom rind

Transverse Cut

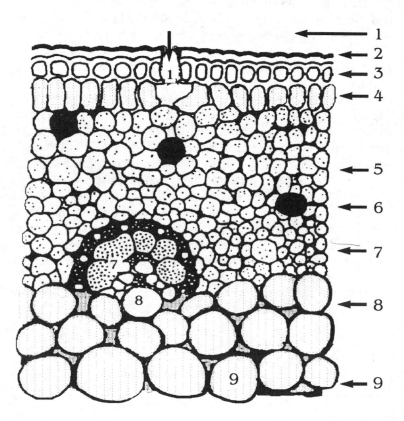

1 - Stomates
2 - Cuticle
3 - Epiderma
4 - Palissadic tissue
5 - Exterior parenchyme
6 - Crystals of calcium oxalate
7 - Pericyclic cells containing the yellow red sap (aloin)
8 - Transverse liaison of vessels
9 - Viscous parenchyme (pulp) which contains the active gel.

Document graciously communicated by Donesta Promotion – Nyon (Suisse)

THE CHEMICAL COMPOSITION OF ALOE VERA

Below we list the elements which have been found in the leaves of aloe vera by general individual elements within general categories, along with an indication of their known medicinal virtues. Most have been identified over the past 50 years.

A) Lignin, saponins, anthraquinones

Aloin : cathartic* and emetic*.
Barbaloin (barbaloin glycoside) : antibiotic* and cathartic.
Isobarbaloin : analgesic* and antibiotic.
Anthranol
Anthracene
Aloetic acid : antibiotic.
Aloe amodine : bactericide and laxative.
Cinnamic acid : detergent, germicide and fungicidal.
Ester of cinnamic acid : analgesic and anaesthesic.
Ethereol oil : tranquilizing.
Chrisophanic acid : fungicidal (skin fungus).
Aloe ulcine : inhibits gastric secretions.
Resistanol

The "Lignins" penetrate the skin easily but their medicinal virtues are little know. The "Saponins" discovered by Wasicky and Hoehne are heterosides (glucides) with well known antiseptic and saponific actions. The "anthraquinones" are known for their laxative and analgesic action. During the past ten years many researchers have confirmed these qualities and the fact that they are non-toxic.

B) Vitamins [12]

Vitamin A (carotene)
Vitamin B1 (thiamine) : Necessary for growth of tissues and the production of energy.
Vitamin B2 (niacine and riboflavine) : act with B6 in the production of blood.
Niacinamide (niacine) : regulator of metabolism.
Vitamin B6 (pyridoxine) : as vitamin B2.
Vitamin B12 (cyanacobalamine) [13]: energy factor in the nutritive functions of the body.
Vitamin C (ascorbic acid) : along with vitamin E it combats infection, helps healing and helps maintain a healthy skin.
Vitamin E (tocopherol) : see vitamin C.
Choline (vitamin of the B complex) helps metabolism.
Vitamin M (folic acid) (vitamin of the B complex) : helps in the formation of blood.

C) Minerals

Aloe contains over 20 minerals, all of which are essential to the human organism.

Calcium : in association with phosphorus, bone growth.
Phosphorus : in association with calcium, bone growth.
Potassium (potassium sorbate).
Iron : works with hemoglobin in the fixation of oxygen.
Sodium
Chlorine
Manganese : in association with magnesium helps maintain

(12) *Vitamins A, C and E are added to aloe vera gel during the stabilization process.*
(13) *Theoretically, vitamin B12 is not found in plants, but is found only in animal food products, and it is known that vitamin B12 is produced in the intestin. In recent years several researchers have found small amounts of it in the gel of the aloe vera plant.*

36

the muscles and nervous system in good order.
Magnesium : (see manganese).
Cooper
Chromium : helps the activity of the enzymes of fatty acids.
Zinc : stimulates the proteins in the healing process.

D) Mono and polysaccharides

Cellulose – Glucose – Mannose – Aldonentose
Uronic acid (Hexo) **– Lipose – Aliinase**
L-rhamnose
Acemannon *(14)*

E) Essential Amino Acids

Amino acids are proteins which furnish energy , act as catalysts (notable in hydrolysis), regulate chemical equilibrium and take part in tissue regeneration.

The human body contains 22 amino acids, 8 of which are so called "essential" because our organism cannot fabricate them. Aloe vera contains 7 of these 8 amino acids, and 11 of the 14 so called "secondary" amino acids which our organism synthesizes from the 8 essential amino acids :

Isoleucine – Leucine – Lysine – Methionine - Phenylalanine – Theonine – Valine

F) Secondary Amino Acids

Asparitic acid – Glutamic acid
Alanine – Argine (or arginine) – 1/2 Cystine
Glycine – Histidine – Hydroxiproline
Proline – Serine – Tyrosine

(14) Numerous researchers around the world are studying aloe and new discoveries are made each year. One of the most recent is acemannon which apparently reinforces the immune system of cancer and AIDS patients. (See page 23 and its note).

G) Enzymes*

The oxidizing enzymes of aloe reduce the basic elements.

Phosphatase - Amylase
Bradykinase or Bradykininase : analgesic, anti-inflammatory, stimulates the immune system.
Catalase : prevents the accumulation of oxygenated water in the system.
Cellulase : facilitates the digestion of cellulose.
Creatine phosphokinase : muscular enzyme.
Lipase : facilitates digestion.
Nucleotidase
Alcaline Phosphatase
Proteolytiase or protease : hydrolyses proteins into their constituent elements. Aloe also contains salicylic acid, chrysophanic acid and volatile oils. Researchers will most certainly discovery other elements in the near future. [15]

---

(15) To learn more about the chemical composition of aloe vera, read :
Robert Dehin, Docteur Aloès.

SOME MEDICINAL ALOE PLANTS

Aloe Succotrina

In ancient times this aloe from the island of Socotra was know throughout the ancient world. The powder of this plant was sold by arab merchants throughout the Mediterranean and as far east as China. It was highly prized for centuries for its therapeutic and magic virtues.

Aloe Vera (Linne) Barbadensis (Miller) or Vulgaris.

In the seventeenth century, the English developed the production of aloe on the West Indies island of Barbados.

The plant was dried and the powder commercialized as a laxative. This industry collapsed when the dutch colonists of South Africa introduced a cheaper product made from the local aloe plant.

There exist two varieties of aloe vera (barbadensis) : a green and a blue. The leaves of the so called green variety have a bright yellowish green color adorned with clear spots. The plant begins to form shoots after the first year and is best for medicinal purposes during its fourth or fifth year.

In the so called blue variety the leaves have a dark bluish green color. This variety matures more rapidly. It reaches maturity during the third year at which time the first shoots also appear.

The two varieties have the same therapeutic virtues.

Aloe africana (Cap aloe).

The Cap aloe and its cousin Curacao aloe, cultivated by the dutch colonists, was until recently the most widely sold aloe. It was commercialized in the form of a powder. It has gradually been surpassed by aloe vera.

Aloe ferox

Along with aloe saponaria this aloe is the most appreciated in the Far East. The Japanese, Chinese and Taiwanese use large quantities or it. They eat it both raw and cooked, drink the pulp after filtering and flavoring it, and use it extensively as a medicine. Today, the Japanese are the largest consumers of both aloe ferox and aloe vera.

Aloe arborescens

This aloe which grows wild in the vast semi-desert regions of southern USSR is the most used by the russian people and researchers. It's medicinal properties were extensively studied and described by the ophthalmologist Vladimir Filatov and the biologist Israel Brekhman.

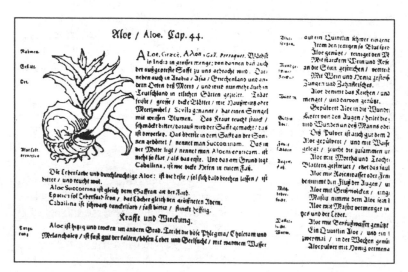

DIFFERENT USES
OF ALOE

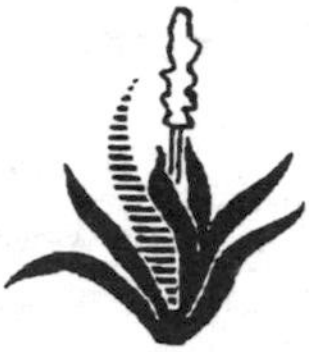

T he pulp (gel) of Aloe can be utilized in several different ways both internally and externally. It is ideal as a first aid treatment of burns, irradiation, sun burns and minor wounds. It is a good haemostatic* and disinfectant.

External Use :

The fresh pulp from the leaf of an aloe vera plant is ideal for external use but a plant is not always available. Fortunately today there exist on the market excellent products containing up to 98% pure pulp of aloe vera. It disinfects and heals wounds.

The pulp of aloe vera is also used in a bio-stimulated version in subcutaneous injection. *(See Wirth : Heal with aloe).*

Internal use :

Liquid aloe vera as a drink is an excellent regulator of the intestines and an excellent food supplement containing numerous vitamins and minerals.

Aloe vera is known to facilitate digestion. It activates blood and lymphatic circulation, and kidney, liver and gall bladder functions , and it alleviates arthritic and rheumatic pains.

Burns :

It is probably in the treatment of burns where aloe vera has shown the most spectacular results. This is best shown by the results of a study made by doctors Martin C. Robson and John

P. Heggers of the Chicago Burn Center : *"whether it be burns caused by fire, cold, hot water, electricity or radiation, aloe relieves the pain, prevents infection and avoids complications"*. In fact it is the ability of aloe to aid in the regeneration of irradiated tissues which has made the reputation of aloe as a miracle plant in both the USA and USSR.

Liver Infections :
The gel of stabilized aloe vera when drunk acts as a remedy against liver infections. It improves the liver functions and is an excellent antidote in case of excessive ingestion of alcohol. It is recommended as a preventative of cirrhosis of the liver.

Stomach and Intestines :
The pulp of aloe vera aids in the prevention of stomach ulcers, facilitates digestion and intestinal transit.

Arthritis, Rheumatism, Back Pain :
Baths* of aloe alleviate the pains of arthritis and rheumatism. Certain therapists recommend light massages of the painful area with the gel or a salve of aloe vera .

Dermatology :
Aloe vera is used widely in dermatology. It is reputed to be effective in the treatment of seborrhea, herpes, red spots, psoriasis, eczema, mycosis and fever blisters.

Allergies :
It is proven that the pulp of aloe vera relieves the itching due to allergies and insect bites, as well as aiding in the healing, in both man and animals.

HYGIENE AND COSMETICS

Today, the cosmetic industry is the second largest in the world, just behind the food production industry. The products offered cover a wide range : lotions and creams of all kinds, shampoos, deodorants, toothpaste, hair-sprays, soaps, bubble-baths, eye washes, powders, lipstick, cleansers, astringents, emollients, moisturizers, beauty masks, and many, many more.

In just a few decades, aloe, already reputed for its medicinal properities, has become widely used in cosmetics. Aloe vera contains many active compounds,including numerous vitamins and minerals, and is known as an astringent, moisturizer and cleanser. It softens the skin, diminishes wrinkles, and cures acne, red spots and many skin irritations. It protects the skin against pollution and is ideal for the treatment of sunburn.

It is no surprise then, that this sector of activity has become an eldorado for cosmetic companies around the world. So, today we can find on the market the best, the useless, and the worst of products, especially the worst. In United states, this phenomenon is called *"the great American cover-up"* or the great camouflage. For, instead of correcting or curing, most of these so called miracle products simply camouflage the problems of the skin and hair.

Of course, aloe vera products are part of this great bluff. Not all products based on aloe vera are of acceptable quality. So a discerning user must judge and compare. The user must also realize that beautiful skin and healthy hair are not acquired overnight by a miracle product. Even with a good and proven product a successful treatment is the result of using the proper products and proven methods over a long period of time. The best products are those manufactured according to pharmaceutical standards which are more rigid than those imposed upon cosmetic products. Below are a few examples of cosmetic uses of a proven quality product.

Skin care
Aloe vera is an excellent astringent and humidifier, and is rich in vitamins and minerals. It is used widely in cosmetics. It is ideal for fragile skins. Skin treated with aloe vera becomes soft and smooth. It accelerates the removal of dead skin and the renewed growth of skin cells. It is ideal for the treatment of sunburns, irritations, red spots, and acne.

Scalp and hair care
When massaging the scalp with aloe vera, the astringent action closes the pores but the penetrating capability of aloe vera fortifies the roots. Shampooing with an aloe based shampoo revitalizes drab and dry hair.

Mouth and teeth care
The many properties of aloe vera make it ideal for mouth and teeth care. Using a daily mouth wash of aloe, and alternating daily brushing with a dental cream with an aloe base and another a fluorine base, helps maintain healthy gums and teeth.

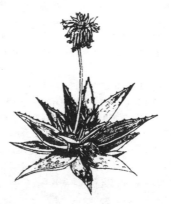

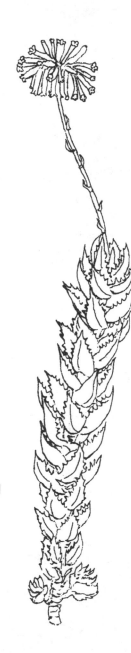

HOUSEHOLD RECIPES

Cuts, Wounds, Bites Burns, scratches

Wash the wound with hot water and soap then coat the surface with pure aloe vera pulp or cover with a gauze saturated with the pulp. Repeat for several days.

Blisters

Prevention : apply a prepared salve of aloe vera or the fresh pulp of a plant to the affected area.

Well formed blister : break the skin with a sterilized needle and fill it with aloe vera pulp. Cover with a gauze.

Burst blister : clean and disinfect the blister, then apply the pulp of aloe vera. After a few moments cover with a gauze.

Sprains, Strains Lumbago, luxation, tendinitis

First place an ice pack on the painful part then cover the area with pure aloe vera gel.

Athletes have developed a special way which consists of freezing the pulp of aloe vera in a paper cup then rubbing the affected area with the frozen pulp and rollng back the paper as it melts.

Chapped Hands

Coat the chapped hands lightly with the gel of aloe vera three times per day.

Mouth Care

To treat bleeding of the gums and mucus : brush the gums gently with a soft brush covered with a mixture of aloe vera pulp and honey.

Skin Problems,
Eczema, mycosis

Cover the affected parts with pure aloe vera gel three times per day.

Falling Hair

Mix the pulp of fresh aloe vera with sweet white wine and massage the scalp regularly with the mixtures. Shampoo regularly with an aloe vera based shampoo.

Dandruff

Massage the scalp regularly with the pulp of aloe vera and wash your hair each day with an aloe vera based shampoo.

Anxiety, Nervous Tension, Stress

The pulp of a fresh leaf or the gel of properly stabilized aloe vera is an excellent health drink and nutritional compliment for anxious, nervous and stressed individuals. A small glass taken before each meal will help them find a new equilibrium and give them the energy to surmount their difficulties.

Tired Eyes

To soothe tired and painful eyes, a few drops of aloe vera eye lotion work wonders. Certain doctors claim that aloe vera is effective in the treatment of more severe eye problems such as cataract and conjunctivitis. But be careful, don't use just any product !

TREATING ATHLETES

Trainers and doctors responsible for the health and treatment of injuries sustained by athletes have learned to use the gel of aloe vera. Application of the gel of aloe vera is effective against blisters, skin scratches, turf burns, and even against odors due to perspiration. It is ideal for the first aid treatment of sprains, strains, tendonitis, dislocations, hygroma, and lumbago. The first virtue of aloe vera is its ability to immediately relieve the pain. The second is its ability to accelerate the healing proccss. Recent discrete research has revealed that due to the nutritive and analgesic powers of the pulp of aloe vera, athletes who drink it improve their performance and it is not detectable in anti-doping tests.

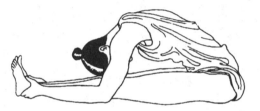

Here are some interesting examples taken from some medical publications :

Doctor Jonathan B. Irving of Chicago treated several hundred athletes with stabilized aloe vera for affections such as : sunburn, lacerations, contusions, sprains, tendonitis, hygroma, and muscular spasms. He then compared the results with those obtained using standard pharmaceutical products. The comparison critera were: reduction of pain, reduction of swelling, improvement of mobility, anti-inflammatory action, and time required to complete the cure. In all cases he had results which were as good or better with aloe vera than with other well known products. In no cases did he find a toxique reaction.

47

Aloe the health and healing plant

In 1992, doctor David E. Cormak published a report in the California medical bulletin concerning the treatment with stabilized aloe vera of 200 cases of scratches, 75 cases of contusions, 80 cases of hygroma, 65 cases of tendinitis, 120 cases of sprains, and 250 cases of arthritis. In all the cases, using the criteria cited in the paragraph above, he obtained results which were as good or superior to those obtained by the use of other current pharmaceutical products.

Doctor Pedro Villa, a Florida surgeon specializing in the treatment of athletes, tested the use of stabilized aloe vera in 80 cases of severe sunburn, 50 cases of contusions and cuts of various types, 30 cases of haematoma, 40 cases of myocitis, and 20 each of tendinitis and hygroma. He reported excellent results concerning the reduction in muscular and articular pain, and the reduction in time required for the healing of wounds and burns.

Gregory Grigorenko, a well known russian trainer, who is an adept of the use of biogenic stimutors of Filatov based upon aloe arborescens in treating his athletes, explains his use in the following terms :

"Aloe used in its bio-stimulated injectable form gives fantastique and rapid results in the treatment of: contusions, and sprains and strains of muscles and tendons. These products are also effective in the treatment of burns and infections due to ingrown nails or atheletes foot.

I use the pure gel of aloe in my treatments by hot and cold baths. I apply the gel immediately to treat contusions, sprains and strains, and I find that the gel rapidly reduces the swelling.

The gel from the leaves of aloe conserved for 10 days in a refrigerator and unexposed to light, proves to be ultra penetrating, thus it quickly transports the active ingredients of aloe to the affected region."

There are dozens upon dozens of such reports by doctors and trainers, especially in the United States and Russia. Little wonder then why the use of aloe vera products by doctors, and trainers for the treatment of top flight athletes and champions has become common practice in the United States and Russia.

ALOE VERA IN VETERINARY MEDICINE

Since the seventeenth century, the British and the Jamaicans prepared, used and exported a product with an aloe base which they called "Horse Aloe". In the United states, in recent years the use of aloe vera in the treatment and feeding of many domesticated animals (dogs, cats, horses, cows, hogs, etc) has become commonplace.

Doctor Richard Holland of the faculty of veterinary medicine of the University of Minnesota states: *"Aloe vera constitutes one of the treatments having the most universal curative properties that I have ever found"* [16].

Due to the continued degradation and pollution of the environment by the modern methods of intensive cultivation and feeding, many producers in the United States are returning to the traditional and more biological ways of raising and caring for animals and plants. The pulp of aloe vera has become one of natural products now being used by many veterinarians in the treatment of a wide variety of injuries and illnesses encountered in the many animals in their care.

For example, in the treatment of horses excellent results have been obtained using aloe vera as a treatment for a wide variety of problems: cuts, puncture wounds, coronet injuries, scaroids, strains and sprains, founder, sore throat, etc.

Excellent results have also been obtained in the care of dogs. A few examples are: seborrhea, ringworm, mange, wounds, allergic dermatitis, lick granuloma, ear infections, and insect bites.

(16) Read : Bill Coats & Richard Holland : Animals in our care.

Some Striking Examples
of Treatment with aloe

Mrs. M.M. of Kingsland, Texas had a dog with an allergy to some grasses which caused red spots on his belly. The itching made him scratch constantly thus making the condition worse. She began a treatment with a gel of aloe vera by rubbing the area thoroughly several times each day. She noticed that the aloe gave the dog almost instant relief from itching. After four days of treatment the red spots were gone and in three weeks the hair had grown back.

In 1975, doctor Robert Northway of Van Nuys, California published a report on his use of aloe vera gel products in his treatment of 42 dogs, 28 cats and 4 horses. He treated them for ailments such as: ringworm, otitis, atopy, and miscellaneous fungi. In 72 of the 74 cases treated, he found the aloe vera products as good as or superior to any other modality available. He also found it excellent in the treatment of tendinitis and inflammation of the joints commonly encountered with race horses.

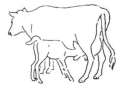

Certain dairy farmers in the USA add aloe vera juice to the drinking water of their cows. To their great surprise they noted that the cows always preferred drinking from the tank containing the aloe. Even more surprising were the results of a study made by Mr. Harriman, of North Dakoda. Over a period of one year he added aloe vera to the drinking water of his 50 cows. He noted a mean monthly increase in milk production of 2000 liters (40 liters per cow).

SCIENCE
CONFIRMS TRADITION

Athletics

At the 1976 Olympic games in Montreal, Canada, after the preliminary trials, four Russian athletes had severe muscular strains and sprains as well as elongations of the Achilles heal.

The anti-doping rules made it impossible for their doctor to administer medications which would give them a chance in the finals. The treatment allowed had no effect and time was short. They began to realize that except for a miracle they had no chance of winning medals in several disciplines.

At that point, the therapist and official trainer for the teams at the University of Texas, offered to help by treating them with a natural salve based upon a plant he did not name. The treatment was successful and three of the Russian athletes won gold metals.

The salve was made of the pure pulp of aloe vera, which is used widely in America in the care and treatment of athletes.

(J.N.M. - F.F.A.)

The Amputation

In his book *"The Silent Healer"* Bill C. Coats recounts the following incident: "October 1975, Dallas, Texas. Dr. David K. Selby entered the doctors lounge, a discouraged man. He

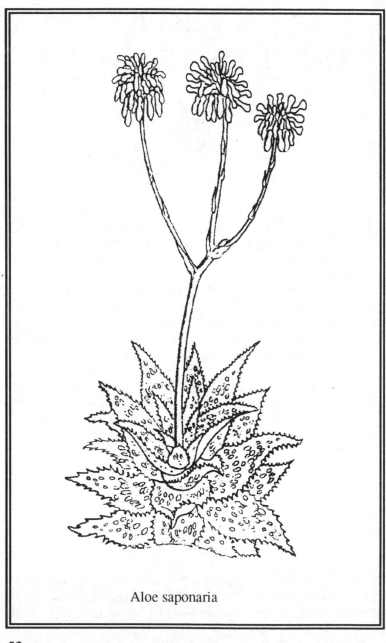

Aloe saponaria

had just completed his sixth operation to remove a severe proteus infection in the calf-bone (tibia) of a teen-age boy's leg. The prognosis: bleak. If the post-operative results were no better than the five preceding, the infection would continue to spread unchecked, and Dr. Selby would have to go in for yet another operation.

The young man had been in a car-bike accident a few weeks earlier that had been serious enough to require the amputation of his left foot. all had gone according to schedule and the customary antibiotics prescribed to avoid secondary infections.

The antibiotics had failed: the leg was suffering a rampant proteus infection. Dr. Selby had prescribed a new series of antibiotics, but those too fell short of stopping the infection. Eventually every known serial antibiotic had been used to try and stem the infection and everyone failed. The operations were a last resort. Selby was at a cul de sac.

I happened to be present in the doctor's lounge when Dr. Selby came in relating his frustrations with the case.

"We've tried every known antibiotic, and nothing works," he said. *"I've operated six times on the boy, going higher on the leg each time. And it's still infected. When I get to his hip, he dies..."*

I told him of the remarkable success other doctors had experienced using our Aloe 99 Gel to fight infections, and showed him some of our bacteriological data to back it up. He was impressed with what he saw, but still remained concerned about possible toxicity, a reservation soon put to rest by two physicians, who had used the Aloe Vera Gel. They told him that they had treated several cases with the Gel and had never experienced a single case of side effects or contraindications.

At this point Selby realized he had nothing to lose. Within a short period of time, he stabilized the boy's leg and inserted a tube into the bone using the 100% Stabilized Gel as a drip. Within a few hours, the proteus infection appeared dormant. In less than forty-eight hours the infection had been eliminated entirely.

The boy recovered, and though fitted with an artificial limb, is healthy and active today."

The Experiment of
Doctor Om Prakash Agarwal

In 1984, a Hindu doctor, Om Prakash Agarval, presented a paper at the convention of the International College of Angiology held in San Antonio, Texas which caused a bit of a sensation. He announced the results of a research he had conducted concerning the benefits of aloe vera on the cardio-vascular system. The study concerned 5000 patients over a period of five years.

His study showed that is was possible to diminish the severity of anginal crises by a factor of 85% by adding the pulp of fresh aloe vera leaves to the daily diet of patients suffering from cardio-vascular problems caused by arteriosclerosis (hardening and clogging of the arteries by fatty deposits). He also noted a significant reduction of the levels of cholesterol and triglycerides in the blood of the patients, as well as an increase in the high density lipoproteins (the good cholesterol).

All these factors contribute to the reduction of the risks of heart attacks. He also found that the aloe vera diet also reduced the blood sugar level in diabetic patients.

According to doctor Agarwal, all of the 5000 patients treated in this manner survived, and none had shown negative side affects during the entire period of the study.

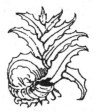

The daily dietary prescription consisted of 100 grams of the fresh pulp of aloe vera plus 20 grams of isabgol (a Hindu medicinal plant known to prevent constipation) mixed with flour to form a kind of bread. *(October 1985). (Medical Gazette, South Texas. Vol.6. N° 50).*

Aloe, Elixir of Long Life ?

After the death of doctor Yernest, a Swedish doctor, at the age of 104, after a fall from his horse, they found among his papers a secret formula for an elixir of long life. The base of the elixir was aloe and the secret formula had been in the family since several centuries. Was it the use of the elixir which explained the longevity of his ancestors? His mother lived to the age of 107, his father 112 and his grandfather 130 !

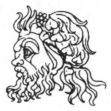

A Cure by Intensive Care

My friend Malcomb Indread of Johannesburg, a former rugby star, was suffering terribly from diabetes. He had grave circulatory complications which he had neglected to treat in time.

One day one of the open sores on his leg became gangrenous and spread to such a point that his doctor was contemplating amputation. Not satisfied with the diagnosis, Malcomb called in his former rugby team trainer, Dr. Robert C. Collins. In spite of the expressed reserve of the hospital medical staff, Collins proposed an intensive cure consisting of external and internal use of fresh aloe vera juice, a plant well known and widely used in South Africa. After three weeks of treatment my friend was out of danger and today, he is playing rugby again, in the senior category.

(Richard Beltram - Capetown).

An Energy booster, pain reliever, and healing stimulator

Dr. Bruce Hedendal, a chiroprator in Boca Raton, Florida, has become an enthusiast of the juice of the aloe vera plant. He first tested the aloe vera juice on himself. *"After a few days of drinking the aloe vera juice, I felt calmer, had more energy, and required less sleep"*, he said. He began to prescribe the aloe vera juice for his patients. They reported sleeping better, feeling less fatigued, and digesting food better. An example: Helen, 83, said: *"may legs seemed to walk by themselves when I walked my four miles each day."*

Dr. James Harrison, a dentist in Lake Worth, Florida, and a friend of Hedendal's, began to drink the aloe vera juice. Not long after he noticed a tremendous increase in his energy and a diminished craving for caffeine and sugar. He soon lost unwanted pounds and the allergy symptoms he had cleared up, and a shoulder pain which he had for two years disappeared. He also uses aloe vera in his dental practice. In some patients undergoing dental surgery, Dr. Harrison irrigates the wound with aloe juice. He finds that the patients have less pain and heal faster.

Stomach and Colon Conditions, and Others

Dr. Lee Cowden, in Dallas, Texas, has observed that a myriad of conditions benefit significantly when treated by oral intake of aloe vera. These include irritable bowl syndrome, ulcerative colitis, esophagitis, peptic ulcer, as well as, rheumatoid arthritis, osteoarthritis, mouth lesions, sore throat, sleep disturbances, and lupus.

Dr. B. Friedlander, a nutritionalist in San Diego, California, has found that patients with chronic colon problems, including constipation, hemorrhoids, colitis and Crohn's disease, benefit from drinking aloe vera juice as part of a nutritional program. He states, *"I notice also that their complexions look better."*

Other Scientific Results

Dr. Robert H. Davis, a physiologist at the University of Pennsylvania College of Podiatric Medicine, has conducted research on aloe since the late 1970's. He says, *"aloe vera contains the greatest number of active substances of any plant I've looked at."*

In laboratory tests on animals, he found that aloe can both prevent and arrest arthritis, improve wound healing, inhibit pain, block inflammation, restore bone growth, and act as a vehicle for the delivery of drugs and nutrients.

In a six month study conducted by a physician (deceased), 29 AIDS patients were given nutritional supplements consisting of aloe vera juice and essential fatty acids, along with their regular diet. Most of the patients with symptoms reported that their energy levels improved within three to five days and all began to gain weight.

At the University of Texas Anderson Cancer Center, researchers have shown that skin cancer induced in mice by exposure to ultraviolet radiation can be prevented or cured by applying aloe vera gel immediately after exposure.

Researchers at the University of Texas Medical Branch and Shriners Burns Center, Galveston, Texas, reported beneficial results when treating burn and frostbite injuries with an aloe vera cream (Dermaide). This cream is also effective in the treatment of: abrasions, minor cuts, electrical burns, mosquito bites, sun burn, and dry itchy skin.

A recent scientific study has shown that an aloe vera plant in a room destroys up to 90% of the formaldehyde, a volitile toxic substance often present in the air of the room. Formaldehyde is a harmful substance introduced into the air by cigarette smoke, paint fumes, insulation, carpet glues and certain food packaging.

It causes irritation of the eyes, nose and throat, and can aggravate the symptoms of asthma.

How to choose
the right products?

In our northern climates, it is not easy to successfully grow aloe vera in the garden or in a pot. So, in our modern world we prefer to buy the products available on the market. But, we must realize that the effectiveness of these aloe vera products depends above all upon the purity of the product, and the method of fabrication and conservation. Today we know that the drying of the pulp of the leaf into a powder destroys most of its therapeutic virtues.

The percentage of aloe vera contained in a particular product as indicated on the label is often misleading. It does not take into account the dilution nor the technique of preservation. You may find on the market a product which has on the label: "100% aloe vera" when in reality it contains only a small amount of a powder of aloe vera diluted in water! Be careful in choosing your products!

Today there are numerous producers of aloe products in numerous countries and several excellent laboratories. But, in order to retain its virtues for a long period of time the products of aloe vera must be properly stabilized. This has proven to be a rather complex and difficult task. However, there are several companies which have succeeded in producing proven and viable products. The best assurance for a buyer today is to be sure that the product has been approved by a serious quality control organization.

Internation Aloe Science Council (IASC)

Ten years ago, the American producers of Aloe formed an association, NASC, to promote the aloe products, control and insure the quality of the products put on the market, and insure that the percentage content of aloe was clearly indicated on the label.

After having developed a test to verify the proportion of aloe vera in a preparation and test the quality, NASC established a system of certification for growers and processors. The first manufacturer to receive authorization for this label was the Texas company "Aloe Vera of America", In 1986, NASC became IASC (international Aloe Science Council) and offers the reputation of its label to serious producers the world over.

Practical Suggestions

Aloe vera is a plant with numerous medicinal properties. Most of its chemical components are known, but not all. Aloe vera contains active molecules which do not necessarily act the same way on everyone and in every circumstance. Even though it is known to be harmless and non-toxic, it does not mean that it can be used without discernment and without following instructions.

It can be used externally and internally. For example, drinking a glass of pure aloe vera juice each day can prove to be an excellent tonic. But in serious cases, even in external use, the treatment should be followed by a competent therapist.

The actual popularity of aloe has resulted in the appearance on the market of hundreds of products. All are not irreproachable, far from it. Many make fraudulent claims. Products made of the powder or concentrate of aloe contain only a relatively small percentage (on the order of 1%) and can in no way be compared to products made of leaf-gel of aloe vera properly stabilized and in concentrations approaching 100%.

These products are on sale in drug stores and health food stores. Some are only available through direct sales. *"Forever Living"*, presently the largest producer and marketer of stabilized aloe vera products, has obtained the label of the IASC, and sells the products in many countries in direct sales by independent distributors.

For those who use the fresh leaf-gel from a live aloe vera plant, the question sometime arises : *"Why doesn't aloe vera always work?"*. The answer is as complex as the plant itself but can be summarized as follows:
– Use of the wrong species of aloe.
– Use of an immature plant or one with degenerated leaves.
– Use of a gel that has been exposed too long, thus neutralized.
– Improper or erratic use during treatment.
– And last but not least, the subtle and unpredictable ways in which it works.

What some famous men have said about Aloe

Mahatma Gandhi
(Letter to Romain Rolland)

"You ask me what were the secret forces which sustained me during my long fasts. Well, it was my unshakable faith in God, my simple and frugal life style, and the ALOE whose benefits I discovered upon my arrival in South Africa at the end of the 19th century."

François -Vincent Raspail
(French chesmist – Carpentras 1794 - Arcueil 1878)

"During the 20 years that I have been treating my patients with aloe, I have found that there are many diseases described by the doctors of antiquity which disappear rapidly when I administer ALOE in the form of granules or powder. Therefore, the good results which I have always obtained, allow me to quote the adage of Roger Bacon :

"Do you wish to live as long as Noah ? Then take some pills of ALOAH!"

Christopher Columbus
(Reported by Salvador de Madariaga)

"Four vegetables are indispensible for the well being of man : Wheat, the grape, the olive, and ALOE. The first nourishes him, the second raises his spirit, the third brings him harmony and the fourth cures him."

VOCABULARY

Aloin : primary active component of aloe found in the resin and powder and identified by Smith and Stenhouse in 1851.

Analgesic : property of a substance to diminish pain by acting on the central nervous system.

Angiosperm : a plant whose ovules are an enclosed cavity (ovary).

Anti-inflammatory : which acts against the inflammation of tissues caused by physical, chemical or biological aggression.

Antibiotic : a plant having the property of slowing down or stopping the development of pathogenic microbes. Ex: aloe, thyme, sage.

Astringent : the property of certain plants to tighten tissues, to stop hemorrhages, diarrhea, etc.

Bactericidal : which has the power to destroy bacteria.

Baths : Immersion of the entire or partial body. A preparation usually of herbal origin added to the bath.

Cathartic : which purifies. a mild laxative.

Cholagogic : a plant which facilitates the flow of bile from the gall bladder to the duodenum. Ex: aloe, mint, olive.

Choleretic : which provokes the secretion of bile.

Collagen : fibrous protein, principal constituent of the inter-cellular substance of conjunctive tissues.

Dermis : conjunctive tissue which together with the epithelium forms the skin.

Diuretic : plant which facilitates the evacuation of water by the kidneys.

Dyspepsy : digestive discomfort and difficulty due to overeating.

Elixir : a liquid preparation usually made of aromatic vegetable substances in alcohol or wine. Often considered to be Magic. Ex: "Elixir of long life".

Emetic : which induces vomiting. Syn. vomitive.

Emollient : which soften, relaxes.

Enzymes : proteins with great catalytic power facilitating the metabolism of molecules produced by the genes.

Fibroplast : cells of conjunctive tissue responsible for the fabrication of collagen fibers which form the skin and muscil tissues.

Fungicidal : which destroys pathogenic fungus causing mycosis of the skin.

Haemostatic : substance which is coagulating and vasoconstricting thus stops bleeding.

Laxative : a substance which facilitates bowel movement, avoids constipation.

Metabolism : the biological and chemical processes which take place in the cells to transform food into energy.

Parenchyme : basic tissues of plants formed of living cells and present especially in the medullary and cortical parts of the stem, leaves and roots. Primary function is the flow of sap.

Phenarogame : a flowering plant which produces seeds.

Placebo : an inactive and inoffensive substance administered to a patient instead of a medicine, usually in the same form and under the same conditions.

Stomatic : a plant which aids the stomach functions.

Virucidal : property of a substance to destroy virus.

BIBLIOGRAPHY

Principal works consulted :

Dr. Emil-August Benz : *Aloe vera Wunderpflanze* Sommerverlag Leipzig.

F. Bloomfield : *Miracle plant Aloe vera* Century Publishing 1985.

Max Brand : *Aloe vera : Die Pflanze der Könige* Berlin 1937.

Père Vittorio Bosello : *Le miracle du Miel et de l'aloès*, in : "Terre Sainte", Couvent St Sauveur, BP. 186 Jérusalem (mai-juin 1994).

Bill. C. Coats & Spanky Stephens : *Healing Winners* Edit. Robert Ahola 1982.

Bill. C Coats : *The silent healer* A modern study of aloe vera (1979).

Bill. C Coats & Richard E. Holland : *Creatures in our care.*
The Vetenary uses of aloe vera (1985).

Robert Dehin : *Docteur Aloès – Aloe vera plante médicinale*
Editions Quebecor Outremont (Québec) Edition française : Laboratoire Marcel Violet, Paris 1992.

Enrique Munoz y Sanchez : *Aloe vera americana* Soledad Mexico.

Robert James : *Aloe vera : nature's miracle plant* Alive Pub. Los Angeles.

Mitsuko Kabuchi : *Aloe vera healing wonder or phantasy ?* Caledonian Press 1986.

Dr. Krumm-Heller : *Magie der Duftstoffe* Verlag Richard Schikowski Berlin.

Vladimir Ladorenko : *Aloe vera and Ayurveda, the science of self healing* Old India Press Bombay.

Lagriffe : *Vieux remèdes du temps* Editions Maloine Paris 1970.

Morissette : *L'aloe vera - Thérapeutique naturelle aux effets universels* in "Médecines Nouvelles" 1989.

Dr. Mutschnick & Dr. Solovieva : *Gewerbetherapie nach der Methode Filatow,* Odessa.

Alexander Popowki : *Auf der Grenze zwischen Leben und Tod* Kultur und Fortschritt Verlag Berlin 1951.

Max B. Skousen : *Manual del Savila "Aloe vera",* Universal Concepts, Huntington Beach, California USA 1980. **Tsunguru Suzuki** : *Aloe Vera* Izuki Osaka 1987.

A.D. Turowa & E.N. Saposchnikowa *Heilpflanzen der UDSSR* Editions Médicales Moscou 1983.

Wolfgang Wirth : *Guérir par l'aloès* Edition Wilhelm Ennsthaler Steyr 1987 (Edition française : Diffusion Soleils).

Werner Zimmermann : *Wunderpflanzen und Gesundheit* Limmat Verlag, Zürich 1936.

TABLE OF CONTENTS

Achevé d'imprimer le 15 avril 1995
sur les presses de la
Nouvelle Imprimerie Laballery
58500 Clamecy (France)
N° d'impression : 504012

ISBN : 2-9508531-1-0
Dépôt légal : avril 1995

Printed in France